Harmony In Connection

How Relationships Shape Our Happiness and Well-Being

By

Kayla Flowers

Disclaimer

Table of contents

Introduction

What does a happy and fulfilled life entail? Is it anything different, like fame, money, or success? Despite the difficulties and changes that come with life, how can we find and keep happiness? For millennia, people have been captivated and confused by these inquiries.

I will share the long-term happiness secrets from the world's longest happiness research, the Harvard Research of Adult Development, with you in this book. This research, which started in 1938 and is still going strong, has tracked the health, employment, families, and general well-being of hundreds of men and women for more than 80 years. Numerous facts and insights into what makes individuals happy and healthy, as well as what influences people's lifespan, have been gleaned from the research.

The study's core finding which may surprise you is that relationships, not money, celebrity, or achievement, are the key to a happy and satisfying life. Our level of pleasure, well-being, and health are significantly influenced by the quality and quantity of our relationships with our family, friends, partners, and community. Strong, sustaining relationships lead to more happiness, better health, and longer lifespans than lonely, isolating, or conflicted lives.

So how can we create and preserve meaningful connections in a hectic and complicated world? In every relationship, there will always be difficulties and disagreements. How do we handle these things?

How can we find time and energy for ourselves and others while juggling our personal and professional lives? How can we change our relationships throughout time and yet develop and adapt?

The most significant and potent source of contentment and well-being in our lives is our relationships. They influence our identity, emotions, thoughts, and behaviors. They can improve our morality, intelligence, happiness, and health. They have the power to instruct, harm, and challenge us. We will examine the science and art of relationships in this book, as well as how they might contribute to a life that is more purposeful and happy. We will also look at how connections differ across cultures, settings, kinds, and domains, as well as how complicated and diverse they are.

Regardless of your age, gender, introversion, or level of marriage, this book will provide you with insightful advice on fostering new relationships and fortifying the ones you currently have at every point in your life. You will not only increase your personal happiness and well-being but also make society a happier and healthier place by doing this.

How to read the book and put its lessons into practice in your own life.

The goal of this book is to be both useful and educational. You will get up-to-date scientific data and analysis on how relationships impact different facets of our happiness and well-being in each chapter. In addition, there are activities, tales, and examples to help you apply the key ideas to your own circumstances.

You have the option to read the whole book or only the chapters that pique your interest. The book may also be used as a resource or a guide if you want some relationship-improvement guidance or inspiration. The book is intended to be a tool to help you identify and maximize your own distinct style and interpersonal potential rather than a one-size-fits-all answer. We hope that after reading this book, you will have a better grasp of both the beauty and power of relationships, as well as a deeper understanding of yourself and others.

Part I

The Science of Relationships.

Chapter 1

The Act of Relationship

A Relationship: What Is It?

Any connection positive or negative between two persons is referred to as a relationship. Relationships with a variety of individuals are possible, including those with family and friends. Even while romantic partnerships are often associated with the term "being in a relationship," it may also apply to a variety of ties one person has with another.

Not every "being in a relationship" entails physical closeness, emotional connection, and/or commitment. Individuals participate in a wide variety of relationships, each with its special qualities.

Fundamental Relationship Types

Most relationships fit into one of the following categories, albeit they don't always match up:

- Family ties
- Ties with friends
- Friends
- Romantic relationships
- Partnerships for sex
- Workplace collaborations
- Situational connections (sometimes referred to as "situationships")

There are other subtypes of relationships within each of these fundamental kinds, and the degree of intimacy in these various forms of relationships may vary substantially. The following are a few of the several relationship types that you may encounter throughout your lifetime.

Relationships may take many various forms, but four basic categories are often recognized: romantic relationships, friendships, acquaintanceships, and familial connections.

- Platonic Bonds: A close, personal tie without either sex or romance is what is known as a platonic relationship. These connections are often characterized by:
  - Intimacy
  - Warmth
  - Gratitude
  - Courtesy
  - Take Care
  - Encouragement
  - Sincerity
  - Acceptance

Platonic relationships may entail friendships between people of the same sex or opposite sex and can take place in a variety of contexts. You could connect with someone in a different context, like a club, sport, or volunteer group you are interested in, or you might develop a platonic friendship with a classmate or coworker.

The social support that this kind of connection may provide is crucial for your overall health and well-being. According to research, having platonic connections may improve your immunity, lessen your chance of sadness or anxiety, and minimize your risk of illness. Platonic relationships are friendships and intimate bonds without sexual activity. Platonic partnerships may sometimes develop into romantic or sexual interactions over time.

✚ Romantic Relationships

Love and attraction for another person are the hallmarks of romantic partnerships. Romantic love may take many different forms, but it often entails emotions of commitment, closeness, and infatuation.

Scholars have devised several terminologies to characterize the experiences and manifestations of love. For instance, according to psychologist Robert Sternberg, love is primarily composed of three things: closeness, decision/commitment, and desire. He defines romantic love as the union of closeness and desire. Over time, romantic relationships often evolve. People usually feel more passionately in the beginning of a relationship. The brain produces dopamine, oxytocin, and serotonin, among other neurotransmitters, during this early stage of infatuation, making individuals feel happy and "in love."

These emotions begin to fade in intensity with time. People become closer and more understanding of one another on an emotional level as their connection grows. In the beginning, romantic partnerships often burn brightly. Over time, sentiments of trust, emotional closeness, and commitment tend to get stronger while the initial intensity of desire typically wanes.

+ Codependent Relationship.

An unhealthy, unbalanced kind of relationship, when one partner is emotionally, physically, or mentally reliant on the other, is known as a codependent relationship.

Additionally typical is the reciprocal dependence of both couples on one another. Both parties have the option to alternately assume the position of caregiver and care recipient. An association that is codependent has the following traits:

- Being the donor and the other person being the taker.
- Going over and above to keep the other person at bay.
- Having the impression that you need permission to accomplish things.
- Being forced to protect or deliver the other person from their own deeds.
- Taking actions that may cause discomfort in order to make someone else happy.
- Feeling unclear about your identity in the relationship.

- Elevating the other person even when they haven't done anything to merit your gratitude or respect.

But not every codependent relationship is the same. The degree of severity might vary. Codependency may affect friendships, romantic partnerships, parent-child relationships, interactions with other family members, and even relationships at work. Codependent relationship are made together. Although one spouse may come out as more "needy," the other partner may really like being needed.

For example, someone who chooses a spouse who is always in need of them may avoid concentrating on their own needs since they feel more at ease being required.

✦ Casual Relationships.

Dating relationships that may entail sex without expectations of monogamy or commitment are sometimes referred to as casual partnerships. Experts contend that the phrase is ambiguous and that various individuals may interpret it in different ways. The authors of research that was published in the Canadian Journal of Human Sexuality state that casual relationships might include the following circumstances:

- One-night encounters.
- Calls from Booty.
- "Sex" partners.
- Friends with benefits.

These kinds of interactions often fall somewhere on a spectrum with respect to the frequency, nature, degree of friendship, and quantity of personal information shared. According to the research, those with more sexual experience than those with less were able to correctly recognize the meanings of these categories.

Among young adults, casual relationships are often prevalent. Casual relationships may have a number of sex-positive advantages as long as they are characterized by consent and communication. Without the emotional strain and energy investment of a more committed relationship, they may satiate the desire for sex, closeness, connection, and companionship. Although they may occur in any age group, casual relationships arc more prevalent in the younger adult population. Communication and consent are essential.

✝ Open Relationships.

One or more parties in an open relationship have sex or have relationships with other people; this kind of consensually non-monogamous partnership is known as an open relationship. In an open relationship, both parties consent to have sex with other people, albeit there could be restrictions or stipulations. Any kind of romantic engagement, whether it be casual, dating, or married, may include open partnerships.

Relationships that are not monogamous are often stigmatized. Nonetheless, data indicates that between 21% and 22% of individuals will engage in an open relationship at some time in their lives.5

Gender and sexual orientation also have an impact on the chances of being in an open relationship.

Men were more likely than women to report having been in open relationships, and those who identify as homosexual, lesbian, or bisexual were more likely to have been in open relationships in the past than heterosexual individuals.

✛ Toxic Relationships.

Any kind of interpersonal interaction when your physical, mental, or emotional health is compromised or in danger is considered toxic. You often feel misunderstood, embarrassed, ashamed, or unsupported in these kinds of interactions.

Relationships of any kind, whether they be sexual, familial, friendship, or professional, may be poisonous.

Relationships that are toxic are defined by:

- Absence of assistance
- Accusing

- Rivalry
- Regulating actions
- Indignation
- Insincerity
- Gaslighting
- Anger
- Envy
- Aggressive but passive behaviors
- Ineffective dialogue
- Ineffective dialogue
- Emphasize

There are instances when poison in a relationship is the result of everyone involved. For instance, if you are always harsh, judgmental, insecure, and pessimistic, you can be adding to the poison. In other situations, one partner in a relationship could act in a manner that engenders negative emotions.

Sometimes this is done on purpose, but other times individuals may not be completely aware of the impact they are having on other people. Due to their prior relationship experiences, which often occurred in their childhood home, they could not be aware of any alternative manner of speaking and behaving.

How to assess your relationship's quality.

Since various individuals may have different perspectives or standards for evaluating a relationship, there is no one right way to determine the quality of your partnership. Still, here are a few methods to evaluate the quality of your relationship:

1. Completing an assessment of relationship quality, such as the one found

at https://www.idrlabs.com/relationship-quality/test.php

2. Using the scale below, the Relationship Assessment Scale

SCALE FOR RELATIONSHIP ASSESSMENT

Citation:

Hendrick, S. S. (1988). A general gauge of relationship contentment. 50, 93–98 in Journal of Marriage and the Family.

Measure Description:

A seven-item questionnaire intended to gauge overall relationship happiness. Each question is answered by the respondents on a 5-point rating system that goes from 1 (poor satisfaction) to 5 (great satisfaction).

Scale:

S/N		Low				High
1	How well does your partner meet your needs?	1	2	3	4	5
2	In general how satisfied are you with your relationship?	1	2	3	4	5
3	How good is your	1	2	3	4	5

	relationship compared to most?					
4	How often do you wish you had gotten into this relationship?	1	2	3	4	5
5	To what extent has your original relationship met your expectation	1	2	3	4	5

6	How much do you love your partner?	1	2	3	4	5
7	How many problems are there in your relationship?	1	2	3	4	5

Items 4 and 7 are reverse-scored.

Scoring is maintained ongoing. The higher the score, the more happy the responder is with his/her relationship.

3. The greatest approach to judging the quality of a relationship is to ask yourself

how you feel about the person you are in a relationship with, how they make you feel, how they treats you, how they satisfy your needs, how they contribute to your happiness, etc.

Ask yourself questions relating to how the relationship has transformed you positively or benefited you positively and how content you are with the new you? The changed you? Or how pleased are you with the aid you receive from your partner?

No matter the connection, whether, family? Casual? Romantic? etc

Access yourself and the influence the connection has on you.

Chapter 2

How relationships affect our physical health and lifespan.

The connections you pick don't simply affect your mental health. The stress or enjoyment they nurture also impacts your long-term and short-term physical health.

Researchers are discovering that the quality of our relationships with our spouses, family members, and friends might be as essential, or in some circumstances, more important, to human health as behaviors like smoking, eating, exercising, and drinking alcohol. Humans are social creatures created to work together toward a shared goal, and, as a consequence, our well-being is strongly related to these ever-important connections.

What Is a Healthy Relationship?

A healthy relationship may vary in how it appears from person to person. However, usually, relationships flourish when couples have open communication, are able to cope with stress effectively together, and are receptive to the views and emotions of their partners.

Health Benefits of a Good Relationship

A vast spectrum of study has

A March 2023 research published in the Journal for Social Psychological and Personality Science tracked 4,005 individuals who submitted check-ins every three days on their blood pressure, heart rate, stress, and coping while also offering ratings of their relationships.

"People with more positive experiences and fewer negative experiences [in their relationships] reported lower stress, better coping, and lower systolic blood pressure reactivity, leading to better physiological functioning in daily life," wrote the research authors.

Additionally, in the United States, marriage is connected to other critical health outcomes that have nothing to do with physiologic stress. For example, our access to health insurance, benefits, tax write-offs, housing, and other essential outcomes are excellent for our health.

Toxic Relationships and Your Health

The flip side of the coin is that bad-quality connections have the opposite impact. Partners that are more negative and angry in their everyday interactions have heightened cardiovascular reactivity, immunological response, greater inflammation as well as higher cortisol levels. Negative relationships produce stress and pressure on the body and may raise the risk of cardiovascular events, and chronic illness and may cause early death.

Impact of poor relationships on physical health:

- Weakened immune system: Chronic stress may depress your immune system, making you more prone to infections and sickness.
- Cardiovascular problems: Negative relationships may raise blood pressure, heart rate, and inflammation, leading to an increased risk of heart disease, stroke, and other cardiovascular difficulties.

- Increased pain perception: Stress and anxiety may heighten pain sensitivity, making current chronic pain disorders worse and perhaps leading to new ones.
- Unhealthy coping strategies: Individuals in unhappy relationships may resort to unhealthy coping techniques including smoking, drinking or drug misuse, and overeating, further compromising their health.
- Chronic illnesses: The cumulative psychological and physical health repercussions of poor relationships might raise the likelihood of acquiring chronic diseases including diabetes, autoimmune disorders, and even some malignancies.

Chapter 3

How relationships affect our mental health and happiness

Our interactions, from deep attachments with family and friends to casual contacts with coworkers and neighbors, have a tremendous influence on our mental health and happiness. They may be a source of love, support, and pleasure, but they can also be a cause of stress, conflict, and misery. Let's investigate both sides of the coin:

The Positive Impact of Relationships.

* Social connection and belonging: Humans are social beings by nature, and feeling connected to others is crucial for our well-being.

Strong connections create a feeling of belonging and community, which helps buffer against loneliness and isolation.

* Support and encouragement: When we confront problems in life, having a supporting network of friends and family may make all the difference. They may give a listening ear, practical aid, and emotional encouragement, which can help us manage stress and bounce back from disappointments.

* Increased self-esteem: Positive connections may increase our self-esteem and confidence. Feeling liked and cherished by others may help us feel good about ourselves and our position in the world.

* Enhanced happiness and well-being: Studies have shown that good relationships are related to improved

happiness, life satisfaction, and general well-being. People with strong social ties tend to have reduced incidences of sadness, anxiety, and other mental health disorders.

The Negative Impact of Relationships.

* Toxic relationships: Unfortunately, not all relationships are pleasant. Toxic relationships, marked by negativity, conflict, and abuse, may have a harmful influence on our mental health. They may lead to stress, worry, sadness, and even physical health concerns.

* Loneliness and isolation: Feeling isolated and alone may be detrimental to our mental health. This might happen if we lack intimate connections, or if our relationships are not rewarding.

* Tension and conflict: Even good relationships may occasionally be a source of tension and conflict. If conflicts are not addressed successfully, they may undermine our relationships and take a toll on our mental health.

Chapter 4

How relationships affect our cognitive talents and creativity.

The subtle dance between relationships and our cognitive capacities and creativity is a fascinating one, with studies demonstrating a complex interaction of both positive and negative effects. Let's look into the unique ways our interactions with people might alter our minds:

Boosting the Brain:

* Social stimulation: Engaging with loved ones, friends, and even strangers keeps our minds engaged and blazing on all cylinders. This frequent connection challenges our thinking, develops our viewpoints, and exposes us to new ideas, all of which may boost cognitive

flexibility, memory, and problem-solving abilities. Think of it as a mental gym where you're always lifting fresh mental weights!

* Emotional well-being: Positive connections give a basis for emotional stability and support. This sensation of safety and belonging decreases stress and anxiety, which may hamper cognitive performance. In a calmer, more optimistic condition, our minds are free to explore, find connections, and think creatively. Imagine your brain as a garden; great connections are the sunlight and rain that enable the flowers of creativity to blossom.

* Shared experiences and learning: Collaborating with people on assignments, participating in fascinating discussions, and just sharing life experiences broaden

our knowledge base and comprehension of the world. This ongoing learning process maintains our brains sharp and adaptive, supporting cognitive development and the capacity to think beyond the box. Think of it as a treasure mine of fresh facts and viewpoints that expand your mental environment.

The Flip Side of the Coin:

* Toxic relationships: Unfortunately, not all relationships are sunshine and rainbows. Conflict, hostility, and emotional abuse may take a toll on our cognitive ability. Chronic stress induced by such interactions may affect memory, focus, and decision-making. Imagine your brain as a stormy sea; toxic relationships are the waves that hurl your ideas about and make it impossible to navigate effectively.

* Social isolation: Loneliness and lack of social interaction may have a harmful influence on cognitive performance. Studies have indicated that social isolation may contribute to cognitive decline, memory loss, and even an increased chance of dementia. Imagine your brain as a lonely flower in a desolate wasteland; without the critical nutrients of social connection, it may wither and struggle to develop.

Chapter 5

How connections affect our moral ideals and social conduct.

How connections impact our moral ideals.

Relationships may alter our moral ideals in many ways, depending on the nature and circumstances of the connection. Moral values are the norms for social existence that control our conduct and influence our actions and reactions. Some moral standards are individualizing, which promotes personal rights and liberties, while others are binding, which controls conduct in groups.

According to the study, individualizing values are not impacted by who we are around, since they are regarded as bad regardless of where and when they occur. For example, we may respect honesty and justice for ourselves and others, regardless matter the scenario or the persons involved. However, binding values are more sensitive to social influence, since they address the moral responsibilities imparted by particular social relationships. For example, we may value loyalty and respect for our family and friends, but not for strangers or adversaries. We may also appreciate authority and tradition for our culture and religion, but not for others.

Therefore, connections might impact our moral values by selectively activating various values in group contexts, according to the needs of the social situation. We may attach greater emphasis to binding values when we are with near others, such as family and friends, than when we are with distant people, such as strangers or acquaintances. We may also alter our moral beliefs to match the expectations and conventions of the groups we belong to or engage with.

Relationships may also alter our moral values by exposing us to new viewpoints and experiences, which can question or modify our moral ideas and judgments. For example, we may learn from our love partner or our co-worker about a new moral value or position that we were not aware of or did not agree with previously. We may also experience a moral dilemma or conflict that compels us to examine or reassess our moral principles and conduct.

How Connections Affect Our Social Behavior

Relationships may impact our social conduct in numerous ways, depending on the kind, quality, and context of the connection. Social behavior relates to how we interact with others, including our verbal and nonverbal communication, collaboration, compliance, hostility, generosity, and group dynamics[1]. Some of the ways that connections might impact our social conduct are:

- Relationships may supply us with social norms, which are the standards and expectations for proper conduct in a specific situation. For example, we may learn from our family and friends how to greet, thank, apologize, or congratulate people. We may also learn from our love partner or our co-worker how to act in various contexts, such as a date or a meeting.

- Relationships may influence our social identity, which is the component of our self-concept that is formed from our participation in a social group. For example, we may define ourselves as a student, a parent, a fan, or a member of a given culture, religion, or race. Our social identity may affect our attitudes, beliefs, values, and actions towards ourselves and others.

- Relationships may affect our social influence, which is the change in our conduct that arises from the actual or perceived pressure from others. For example, we may conform to the beliefs or behaviors of our peers, or we may comply with the requests or demands of our authority figures. We may also convince or be persuaded by others to adopt a given point of view or course of action.

- Relationships may enhance our social skills, which include the capacity to communicate effectively, work with others, settle problems, and control emotions. For example, we may strengthen our social skills by practicing active listening, offering criticism, showing empathy, bargaining, or compromising with others. We may also learn from our role models or mentors how to handle various social settings.

- Relationships may boost our social support, which is the emotional, informational, or material aid that we get from others. For example, we may gain from the social support of our family and friends while we are going through a tough moment, such as a loss, stress, or difficulty. We may also give social assistance to people who are in need, such as by offering comfort, guidance, or aid.

Part II

The Art of Relationships

Chapter 6

The Five Love Languages

You may show love to your significant other often, but do you genuinely take the time to make sure you're conveying it the way your spouse wants to receive it? Even love may often be lost in translation when two lovers speak different love languages.

What are the 5 love languages?

The five love languages are five distinct methods of expressing and receiving love: words of affirmation, quality time, receiving presents, acts of service, and physical contact. Not everyone transmits love in the same manner, and equally, individuals have varied ways they like to receive love.

The notion of love languages was invented by Gary Chapman, Ph.D., in his book The 5 Love Languages: The Secret to Love That Lasts, where he discusses these five diverse forms of conveying love, which he condensed from his expertise in marital therapy and linguistics.

We all may connect to most of these languages, but every one of us has one that speaks to us the most.

"Discovering you and your partner's primary love language and speaking that language regularly may [create] a better understanding of each other's needs and support each other's growth."

Here's a summary of each of the five love languages Chapman describes:

1. Words of affirmation

People with words of affirmation as a love language prioritize verbal acknowledgments of affection, including numerous "I love you's," compliments, words of gratitude, vocal encouragement, and frequently regular digital contacts like texting and social media participation.

Written and verbal demonstrations of love mean the most to these individuals and couples. These expressions help people feel understood and loved.

2. Quality time

People whose love language is quality time feel the most cherished when their spouse actively wants to spend time with them and is always down to hang out. They really enjoy when active listening, eye contact, and complete presence are valued trademarks in the partnership.

This love language is all about providing your complete focus to that one particular person, without the distraction of television, phone displays, or any other outside interference. They have a strong desire to actively spend time with their significant other, holding meaningful talks or enjoying recreational activities.

3. Gifts

Gifts are a relatively clear love language: You feel appreciated when others offer you "visual symbols of love," as Chapman describes it. It's not about the monetary worth but the symbolic concept behind the thing. People with this style realize and cherish the gift-giving process: thorough contemplation, the purposeful selection of the item to symbolize the connection, and the emotional rewards from getting the present.

People whose love language is getting presents like being given something that is both tangible and meaningful. The trick is to offer meaningful items that matter to them and represent their values, not necessarily yours.

4. Physical touch

People with physical contact as their love language feel loved when they get physical expressions of affection, like kissing, holding hands, snuggling on the sofa, and having intercourse. Physical closeness and touch may be immensely encouraging and serve as a strong emotional link for those with this love language. The origins go back to our youth, Motamedi observes, some individuals only felt real care and love by their parents when they were hugged, kissed, or touched.

People who show their gratitude using this language, when they agree to it, feel valued when they are hugged, kissed, or snuggled. They love the sensation of warmth and comfort that comes with physical contact.

5. Acts of service: If your love language is acts of service, you cherish when your spouse goes out of their way to make your life simpler. It's things like bringing you soup when you're ill, making your coffee for you in the morning, or collecting up your dry cleaning for you after you've had a hectic day at work. This love language is for persons who feel that deeds speak louder than words. Unlike those who want to hear how much they're cared for, those on this list desire to be shown how they're

valued. Doing the smallest and major duties to make their life simpler or more comfortable is greatly loved by these folx.

In terms of personal relationships, Acts of Service is a language that may best be characterized as doing something for your spouse that you know they would want, such as filling up their gas, watering their plants, or making them a meal.

When you offer Acts of Service, you give up your time. This non-verbal type of love might be time-consuming and stressful, but if it's what your spouse needs, then it's worth the effort.

When it comes to completing Acts of Service, here are four things you may do:

- Pay attention to the minor things: what your spouse wants to do on your next vacation together, how much sugar your partner puts into their morning coffee, what time your partner's favorite program is on, etc. Take notes, if you can't recall.

- Consider the things your spouse doesn't love doing: If your spouse complains about taking out the garbage, studying financial terms, cleaning the area between the wall and the dresser, or walking the dog, then you may undertake these activities for your partner. If your spouse doesn't enjoy interacting with the cable provider, offer to take on responsibility for the monthly cable payment.
- Focus on actions that are simple for you to incorporate within your schedule: Pay attention to your partner's schedule each week and see if you can put in Acts of Service.

Maybe your spouse has limited time between their exercise in the morning and their first work meeting. Plan to have coffee and breakfast ready and waiting.

- Utilize your talents: If you understand something your spouse doesn't, offer your services. If you're more handy than your spouse, for example, concentrate on handyman jobs like changing your partner's oil, or replacing the broken lighting in the bathroom.

Even if your spouse chooses another love language, Acts of Service may be useful for any healthy relationship. According to 2016 research done by the Pew Research Center, more than half of all married couples agreed that sharing chores was a fundamental necessity in a happy marriage. Whether it's part of your love language or not, it's crucial to make sure that you and your spouse are both content with how much you do around the home.

Receiving Acts of Service

If you like to receive Acts of Service above all other love languages, then it's crucial to inform your spouse of this. Just make sure you are courteous and patient, while you ask for the things you desire. Acts of service aren't always simple to execute, and you shouldn't expect that your spouse will do all you ask just because you like Acts of Service.

Many times, Acts of Service may be a tough love language to adopt, since it needs so much effort, and frequent, preparation. Maybe your companion is studying for their PhD and unable to concentrate on any actions. Maybe your lover arrives home late after another long day of work, just to offer you thirty minutes of quality time without a TV or smartphone. Try to treasure these attempts, realizing that your spouse certainly loves you, even if they can't conduct Acts of Service that day or week.

Love language quiz: What is my love language?

To identify your type, read the following sentences and highlight the ones that profoundly connect with you. Filter it through:

How do you demonstrate love?

What do you complain about in a relationship?

What do you seek or actively require from your relationship on a day-to-day basis?

The one with the most statements you relate to is your major love language. If two or more languages are deadlocked for first place (which is often!), utilize the process of elimination and work your way down the list until you are left with one or two languages that you are not ready to part with.

Words of affirmation quiz

a. You truly prefer hearing your spouse say, "I love you." Those three words are extremely significant, precious, and comforting for you to hear. Again and again and again.

b. You enjoy it when you are being recognized and rewarded. It's good to have your efforts appreciated with pleasant words, no matter how modest it is. It lets you realize that you are cherished. Extra points if it's out of the blue.

c. The details count, and it's crucial your spouse notes on things like whether you changed your hair or really dressed in work clothes instead of your jammies for your Zoom work call. It indicates they are paying attention, which makes you feel valued.

d. You feel cherished when they take the time to carefully consider and remark on something great they perceive you doing.

e. When you do something good for your spouse, they respond, "Thank you," which helps you feel noticed and validated.

Quality time quiz

a. You prefer to spend undisturbed time with your lover. It's vital you have enough time to hang out and appreciate each other with undivided attention. No distractions, please.

b. It's significant when they make time for you, prioritize you in their schedule, and don't cancel plans.

c. Creating memories and memorable times together is incredibly essential. Sharing new experiences means the world to you.

d. Time is precious, and it's vital to take up every second of your time together.

e. You feel pleased and joyful when you are near your lover, even if you aren't actually accomplishing anything. The key thing is you are spending concentrated time together.

Acts of services quiz

a. You feel taken care of when your spouse supports you and helps lessen your duties when they undertake tiny chores or jobs for you. Domestic happiness awakened.

b. It matters a lot when someone follows through on something, particularly if they are paying attention and stepping in to assist. When they do this, you trust your spouse to pay attention to the minor nuances.

c. You believe language is cheap; action matters everything. You need someone to come through and to know you can depend on them. Show, not tell.

d. You enjoy it when your spouse steps in to do simple things for you to make your life easier.

e. If you're feeling worried or exhausted, it would be wonderful if your spouse viewed it as a chance to step up and lessen your load by taking something off your plate that's simple for them to accomplish. That tiny gesture makes you feel taken care of.

Gifts quiz

a. You feel cherished when you get a present. The present itself is lovely, but it's really the idea behind it that counts: The gift becomes an item that lets you remember they were thinking of you, which fills you with affection.

b. After a date or a vacation, it's great to take a keepsake home with you. Seeing the object reminds you of those cherished experiences.

c. The finest presents are the thoughtful ones. If it's a surprise present, even better. It enhances the link and establishes a deeper connection for you.

d. During holidays, birthdays, or anniversaries, you want to recognize it with a gift of some type. such days are extremely special, and you adore utilizing such days as a reminder of your commitment.

e. The act of getting a present communicates that you are recognized, cared for, and cherished. You truly thrive on the care behind the gesture and appreciate nostalgic goods.

You may also Take the Quiz

Take a free love language questionnaire (https://www.verywellmind.com/love-language-quiz-7562463) to find out which love language you relate with the most.

Understanding Your Partner's Love Language

If your favorite language is Quality Time, but your spouse continues concentrating on Acts of Service, then you may feel slighted when your partner spends time washing your vehicle instead of giving you undivided attention. Make sure you and your spouse are upfront about your preferences and find a method to work together to reach the mutually desired outcomes. If your spouse appreciates when you cook, for example, maybe you can start by providing a weekly breakfast for them.

Now we would look at how we might establish healthy relationships by doing the things that matter.

Chapter 6

Developing thankfulness and pleasant feelings in our relationships.

Creating an atmosphere and mentality that actively supports reciprocal recognition, appreciation, and emotional well-being is necessary to cultivate good feelings and gratitude in partnerships. It entails making deliberate attempts to cultivate these emotions and show thankfulness in a variety of ways; it goes beyond just feeling good. This is what it implies:

1. Conscientious Recognition:

- Being aware of and grateful for the good things in the partnership. Acknowledging your partner's or other people's good traits, contributions, and strengths is part of this.

2. Grateful Expressions:

- Make an effort to show your spouse how much you value and appreciate all of their accomplishments, no matter how tiny. This may be accomplished by deliberate gestures, written notes, or spoken words.

3. Effective Interaction:

- Promoting constructive communication by concentrating on the good parts of the situation rather than focusing on the bad. This entails speaking in an encouraging and affirming manner rather than a critical one.

4. Charity Deeds:

- Performing random acts of kindness on a regular basis to show consideration and concern. The general happiness of a partnership may be greatly enhanced by little, kind actions.

5. Generating Satisfying Encounters:

- Engaging in activities that provide satisfaction and delight to both spouses. This might be as easy as exploring new things, spending quality time together, or making happy memories together.

6. Recognizing Success:

- Honoring individual and group accomplishments, anniversaries, and triumphs. In a relationship, acknowledging successes helps to foster a feeling of validation and support.

7. Rituals of Gratitude:

- Forming routines or habits that foster appreciation, such as a weekly reflection on the good parts of the relationship or a thankfulness practice every day. This aids in keeping the good things in mind.

8. A Positive Attitude:

- Developing an optimistic outlook both individually and as a pair. This entails making the deliberate decision to see obstacles as chances for development and to remain upbeat in the face of difficulty.

9. Environment of Support:

- Establishing a setting that promotes candid communication and emotional health. People may express themselves genuinely and have pleasant emotional experiences when they feel protected and encouraged.

10. Sympathy:

- Promoting a positive feedback loop via mutual aid. Reward and happiness spiral out of control when both spouses actively participate in constructive interactions.

11. Gratefulness During Difficult Times:

- Being thankful even in the face of adversity. This entails seeing the bright side of things, expressing gratitude for the qualities that surface throughout hardship, and standing by one another in times of need.

The mechanics of developing thankfulness and good feelings might alter depending on the kind of connection. Here are some customized recommendations for different kinds of relationships:

Romantic Relationships:

1. Open Communication: Promote candid and open dialogue. Regularly share your

thankfulness, show appreciation, and talk about how you're feeling.

2. Date Nights: Plan frequent evenings for yourself to spend valuable time together. This may foster happy memories and preserve the romantic side of the partnership.

3. Surprise gestures: Keep the romance going by giving your significant other tiny presents or kind gestures out of the blue. It might be as easy as writing a romantic letter or as complex as organizing an unexpected weekend trip.

4. Physical Affection: In romantic relationships, physical contact and affection are essential. Show your love for them on a regular basis with hugs, kisses, and other physical affection.

Family Relationships:

1. Family Rituals: Create customs and rituals inside your family. Family rituals, such as movie nights, weekly dinners, and holiday celebrations, foster a feeling of cohesion and joyful anticipation.

2. Verbalize Your affection: Don't presume that your family members are aware of your affection. Tell them you love and thank them for being in your life, using words to convey your gratitude.

3. Support During Difficulties: Be understanding and helpful when things are hard. The family tie is reinforced as members support one another during trying times.

4. Quality Time: Take time as a family to spend together. Playing games, cooking together, or taking walks are examples of

shared activities that make people feel good.

Friends Relationships:

1. Regular Check-Ins: See your buddies on a regular basis. Thank them for their friendship and find out how they are doing.

2. Celebrate Milestones: Honor one another's successes and significant anniversaries. No matter how large or little, feeling good about yourself is enhanced when you recognize and enjoy your achievements.

3. Common Interests: Take part in things that you both want to do. Hobbies in common may create a supportive and joyful atmosphere for your connection.

4. Random Acts of compassion: Show your pals some love and compassion in

unexpected ways. It may be arranging a surprise trip, giving a modest gift, or sending a kind note.

Work Relationships:

1. Recognition: Give your colleagues efforts your acknowledgment. Thank them for their contributions to the group.

2. Good Feedback: Congratulate someone when they do something well. Saying "thank you" is a little but effective approach to fostering nice feelings in the workplace.

3. Team Building Exercises: Take part in exercises that promote teamwork. Colleague connections may be strengthened and a supportive work environment can be created as a result.

4. Collaboration: Promote cooperation and group efforts. A feeling of togetherness

and shared success is fostered when people collaborate to achieve similar objectives.

5. Parent Children Relationships:

Quality Time: Invest time in your child's favorite hobbies by spending quality time with them.

Give your kid encouragement and praise to help them feel more confident and good about themselves.

Set an example of appreciation in your own life and inspire your youngster to follow suit.

6. Long-Term Partnerships:

Regular Communication: Whether via phone conversations, video chats, or texts, stay in touch by communicating on a regular basis.

Surprise Gifts: As a token of your thanks and devotion, send care packages or surprises.

Arrange Visits: Arrange visits whenever you can to build memories and shared experiences.

7. Neighbourly Connections:

Community Engagement: To foster a feeling of belonging, and take part in local events and activities.

Assisting One Another: Provide aid when required and convey appreciation for the help received.

Socialize: Arrange informal get-togethers to foster a sense of community and get to know your neighbors.

Importance

It's important to foster thankfulness and pleasant feelings in partnerships for a number of reasons:

1. Improves Relationship Contentment:

- People feel happier and the emotional bonds between friends, family, and lovers are strengthened when they feel valued and appreciated.

2. Supports Mental Health:

- Gratitude and happy feelings have been connected to better mental and emotional health.

3. Deepens the Emotional Bond

4. Promotes Mutual Exchange:

People are more inclined to return the favor in a relationship when they feel appreciated and happy. As a result, a positive feedback loop is established in which both partners actively contribute to the relationship's success.

5. Enhances Interaction

6. Develops Adaptability:

A thankful and optimistic outlook makes it easier for people and couples to overcome obstacles. A foundation of thankfulness and good emotions may serve as a shield against adversity, encouraging perseverance and a desire to collaborate to solve issues.

7. Increases Dedication

8. Promotes a Happy Environment:

- A pleasant atmosphere in relationships is influenced by positive feelings.

9. Fosters Individual Development

10. Makes Memories That Last:

Chapter 7

How to settle disputes and communicate well in our relationships

How to Have Effective Communication

Effective communication assumes several forms based on the kind of connection you're managing. The following are specific advice for every category:

1. Outsiders:

* Open your body language and grin: An accessible smile and pleasant manner help to break the ice and promote conversation right away.

* Use plain, straightforward language: Steer clear of jargon and extremely complicated wording, particularly when

speaking with someone from a different cultural background.

Ask open-ended inquiries to demonstrate your sincere interest in learning more than just a yes/no response. This starts a dialogue and gives you further information about them.

* Respect personal space: Keep a suitable distance and be aware of local customs around touching.

* Listen intently and strike up a conversation: Demonstrate your curiosity by paying close attention to them and participating in humorous dialogue.

2. Members of the family:

* Adapt your communication style: Take into account the different communication styles that members of your family prefer. While some people may value a more

nuanced approach, others might prefer directness.

* Exercise active listening: Pay close attention to what your family members are saying. Refrain from interjecting and make an honest effort to comprehend their viewpoint.

* Select your moment: Decide on a suitable moment when everyone is composed and open to discussing delicate subjects. Steer clear of contentious topics while the family is together or when emotions are running high.

* Use "I" statements: Make productive use of "I" statements to communicate your wants and emotions. This promotes understanding and helps prevent blaming.

* Acknowledge shared history and traditions: To foster rapport and

connection, make allusions to family lore, inside jokes, or cultural customs.

3. Your Partner:

* Engage in open and honest communication: Be forthright and honest in sharing your needs, wants, and ideas. Establish a safe environment where being vulnerable is valued and encouraged.

* Practice active listening: Pay close attention to what your companion is saying. Try to grasp their point of view as you listen to them objectively.

* Make use of positive affirmations: Consistently show your mate your love and gratitude. Congratulate them on their accomplishments, acknowledge their efforts, and give them support.

* Retain healthy boundaries: Acknowledge and respect one another's

desire for privacy and alone time. Be mindful of your partner's needs and express your limits in a clear and concise manner.

* Participate in cheerful communication: Use humor, inside jokes, and lighthearted conversation to keep things lighter and enjoyable. This keeps the connection lively and develops the bond.

4. Friends:

* Show your pals that you're here for them through thick and thin; be encouraging and supportive. When assistance is required, provide a sympathetic ear, supportive words, and useful advice.

* Retain a cheerful and optimistic demeanor: Be the buddy who makes the group laugh and smile. Be a good role

model for your peers by sharing your own experiences.

* Respect individual differences: Accept the distinct personalities and communication methods of your pals. Refrain from criticizing or attempting to modify their choices.

* Be aware of social media communication: Prioritize in-person conversation over online communication, even if it's more convenient, to build relationships and prevent miscommunication.

* Participate in shared activities: Take time to do something you both like doing as a couple. Friendships are strengthened and enduring memories are created via shared experiences.

Good communication requires mutual understanding. Finding what works best for you and the people in your life is the key; these are simply suggestions. Have patience, engage in active listening, and make it a constant goal to communicate in a courteous and straightforward manner. You may strengthen your bonds and promote greater understanding with everyone you come into contact with by customizing your approach to each interaction.

How to work out disagreements in our relationships

Although managing disagreements may be challenging, finding a good solution can improve your relationships. The following advice is specific to the many kinds of relationships:

1. Outsiders:

* Retain your composure: Refrain from becoming defensive or angry, since this might escalate the issue. Inhale deeply and maintain composure.

* Seek a resolution: If the disagreement is over a little annoyance, such as someone bumping into you by mistake, just say "I'm sorry" or provide a quick acknowledgment of the problem and move on. If it's more severe, try to work out a solution that will cause the least amount of inconvenience to you both.

* Seek help if needed: Do not be afraid to ask for assistance from bystanders or authorities if the confrontation seems dangerous or intensifying.

2. Members of the family:

* Take a break: If emotions are running high, give yourself some space to calm down before tackling the problem. This gives everyone a chance to collect themselves and deal with the problem coolly.

* Find the ideal setting: Look for a quiet area where you can have an honest conversation without interruptions.

* Remain focused on the problem, not the person: Steer clear of blame games and personal assaults. Remain focused on the particular problem at hand and work together to find a solution.

* Empathy and active listening: Make an effort to comprehend the viewpoint of the other person by demonstrating empathy and active listening. Be mindful of their

emotions and worries prior to voicing your own.

* Make concessions and look for common ground: Be prepared to reach an accommodation and come up with a solution that benefits all parties. Recall that disagreements often provide chances for development and comprehension.

3. Your Partner:

* Practice "I" statements: Use "I" statements to effectively communicate your wants and emotions. This promotes understanding and helps prevent blaming. Saying "I feel hurt when you..." as opposed to "You always make me feel..."

* Stop talking about complaints and start fixing problems: Move the discussion away from complaining and toward finding solutions. Collaborate to determine

the main source of the disagreement and come up with solutions.

* Retain a polite tone: Steer clear of screaming, calling names, and other impolite communication techniques. It's important to treat one another with respect, even when there is disagreement.

* Take pauses when necessary: If the discussion becomes hot, stop for a little while to let things settle down before continuing. This gives you time to collect your thoughts and refrain from saying anything you could come to regret.

* Seek professional assistance if needed: If issues are coming up again or you're finding it difficult to work things out on your own, you may want to think about getting help from a therapist or counselor.

4. Friends:

* Take direct aim at the problem: Steer clear of passive-aggressive conduct and don't repress your emotions. Pick a convenient time and location to discuss the matter directly with your buddy.

* Pay attention to understanding: Pay close attention to your friend's viewpoint and make an effort to comprehend their emotions without interjecting. Be sure to acknowledge their perspective before voicing your own.

* Apologize if necessary: If you've made a mistake, own up to it and provide a heartfelt apology. Expressing regret might help to resolve the disagreement.

* Pardon and move on After the matter has been handled and settled, don't think back on previous offenses. To keep your

connection healthy, forgive your buddy
and put the disagreement behind you.

* Seek assistance if needed: Don't be
afraid to ask for help from other friends or
a responsible adult if the disagreement
seems severe or hard to handle.

Conflict resolution is a talent that requires
patience and practice. Be prepared to
make concessions, speak honestly and
freely, and ask for assistance when
required. You may improve the quality of
your relationships and the ties you have
with the people you care about by
handling disagreements constructively.

Chapter 8

Supporting and nurturing each other goals.

Relationships of any kind need partners to encourage and support one another's development and aspirations. Depending on the kind of relationship romantic, family, friendship, or professional the strategy may change. Here are some broad principles for encouraging and fostering development in many kinds of relationships:

1. Romantic Connections:

- Communication: Be candid while discussing your own objectives. Make certain that each partner feels understood and heard.

- Shared Goals: Establish shared objectives and collaborate to achieve them. This promotes a feeling of cohesion and a common goal.

- Support: Express words of support and acknowledge one another's accomplishments. Provide inspiration when things become hard.

- Respect Independence: Give yourself room to develop yourself. Acknowledge and respect each other's need for personal goals.

2. Family Connections:

- Quality Time: Make the most of your time together by creating a caring and encouraging atmosphere.

- Open Communication: Promote candid dialogue among family members. Discuss goals, difficulties, and advancements.

Collaboration: Work together on initiatives and objectives as a family. This may enhance the feeling of achievement and community.

- Empathy: Show compassion for one another's hardships and provide emotional support.

3. Romantic Relationships:

- Active Listening: Pay close attention to the goals and struggles of your friends by actively listening to them.

- Offer Assistance: Help them reach their objectives by offering your resources or expertise when required.

- Celebrate Achievements: Honor the victories of your friends and support them when they face obstacles.

- Honesty: Give truthful comments and, where needed, give helpful criticism.

4. Associations in the Profession:

- Mentorship: Form connections between mentors and mentees to support career advancement.

- Team Collaboration: Encourage a cooperative workplace where team members may assist one another in achieving their professional objectives.

- Recognition: Honor and commemorate accomplishments in the workplace. This fosters an inspiring and upbeat work environment.

- Training and Development: Promote and assist in continuous education and skill improvement.

5. Relations between parents and children:

- Encouragement: Give the child's interests and abilities encouragement and positive reinforcement.

- Education: Encourage learning and assist individuals in pursuing their interests.

- Role Modeling: Set a good example for them by acting out the morals and virtues you want them to acquire.

- Open Dialogue: Keep lines of communication open in order to comprehend and address their goals and issues.

General Advice

- Empathy: Recognize the thoughts and emotions of the other person.

Patience: Realize that obstacles are a normal part of the learning process and that personal development takes time.

- Adaptability: Adjust to evolving objectives and desires with flexibility.

- Collaboration: When feasible, work with others to achieve shared goals.

The secret to every relationship is to cultivate an atmosphere of mutual respect, trust, and support. The effectiveness of these initiatives is greatly influenced by consistent communication and a sincere concern for the other person's welfare.

Chapter 9

Handling difficulties and setbacks in your relationships.

Difficulties and Solutions for Various Relationship Types:

1. Outsiders:

Difficulties:

* Establishing trust and connection: It's challenging to establish a close bond with someone you don't know well.

* Overcoming shyness and social anxiety: Striking up a conversation with a stranger might be intimidating.

* Managing cultural differences and misinterpretations: Diverse backgrounds might lead to misinterpretations.

Solution:

* Begin with tiny gestures: A kind wave, grin, or deed of assistance may create a connection and break the ice.

* To establish rapport, actively listen and demonstrate genuine interest by asking open-ended questions and paying close attention to what is being said.

* Look for chances to exchange experiences: Join groups, take part in activities, or volunteer with others to discover areas of agreement.

* Respect cultural differences: Learn about their traditions and steer clear of presumptions.

2. Members of the family:

Difficulties:

* Differing values and expectations: Conflicting expectations and opposing points of view may arise in family relations.

* Unsolved grudges and prior issues: Long-standing grievances and unsolved disputes may come up again.

* Misunderstandings and communication problems: It may be difficult for families to communicate clearly and honestly with one another.

Solution:

* Exercise open and honest communication: Make use of "I" statements, concentrate on finding solutions, and actively listen to other people's points of view.

* Establish healthy boundaries and respect limits: Make sure you express your

demands clearly and provide personal space.

* * Let go of grudges and move forward from previous hurts: Resentments impede growth. Make the decision to forgive and concentrate on creating a bright future.

* Seek professional assistance if necessary: To resolve ingrained problems or impasses in communication, think about family therapy or counseling.

3. Partners:

Difficulties:

* Maintaining emotional closeness and connection: Routines and diversions may wear down an emotional relationship over time.

* Managing disparities in needs and communication styles: Misunderstandings and animosity may result from clashing communication styles.

* Managing life transitions and unforeseen obstacles: Outside variables like sickness or job loss may put the partnership to the test.

Solution:

* Make meaningful talks and quality time a priority: Plan frequent date evenings, participate in hobbies together, and pay attention to each other.

* Empathize and comprehend: Make an effort to grasp your partner's point of view and give voice to their emotions.

* Be willing to make concessions and work together to discover solutions:

Cooperate to identify solutions that benefit you both.

* Ask for professional assistance if necessary: Couples counseling may be a helpful tool for resolving conflicts and overcoming communication obstacles.

4. Friends:

Difficulties:

* Life changes and divergent interests: People might drift apart as a result of priorities and interests changing as they mature and develop.

* Misunderstandings and resentments: Unspoken expectations or unresolved disputes may harm a friendship.

* Preserving equilibrium between personal lives and the relationship: It's essential to strike a balance between fostering

friendship and fulfilling personal obligations.

Solutions:

* Express yourself honestly and openly: State your wants and sentiments while addressing any problems in a courteous and straightforward manner.

* Retain frequent communication and make an effort to remain in touch: Arrange gatherings, give each other regular calls or texts, and keep each other informed about one other's activities.

* Respect personal needs and boundaries: Recognize that friends have varying needs and priorities, and give each other room when necessary.

* Be receptive to reestablishing contact and doing new things: Rekindle the

relationship by venturing into unfamiliar territory and regaining common ground.

Chapter 10

How to acknowledge and cherish the pleasures and advantages of our relationships

.

Our happiness and well-being depend on our relationships since they may provide us with friendship, emotional closeness, social support, and personal development1. The following are a few ways we might acknowledge and enjoy the pleasures and advantages of our relationships:

- Show your gratitude: Gratitude is the attitude of admiration and thanksgiving for the things in life that we consider important or worthwhile. Experiencing gratitude may lead to increased happiness, health, and relationship satisfaction·4.

Gratitude may be shown to partners, family, friends, and even complete strangers via presents, messages, praises, and "thank you" notes. Another way we might cultivate thankfulness is to jot down our daily blessings in a gratitude notebook.

- Share happy memories: Recounting happy memories with others may make us happier and strengthen our relationships and mutual trust. Anything that makes us feel good might be considered a positive experience, including a well-written joke, stunning scenery, a delectable meal, or a personal victory. Positive experiences may be spread to others by telling them about them, letting them see images or videos of us, or even asking them to come along.

- Honor major events and successes in your life: birthdays, anniversaries, graduations, promotions, and awards are examples of milestones and achievements. Joining others in celebrating life milestones and accomplishments may help us feel better about ourselves and express our gratitude for their contributions and hard work. We may hold a party, send a card, make a toast, or give a speech to honor others' milestones and accomplishments.

- Enjoy yourself and have fun with others: Having fun and enjoying ourselves with others may make us happier and help us make wonderful memories and feelings with them. Anything that makes us happy may be done with others to have fun and enjoy each other, including playing games, watching movies, taking excursions, or engaging in interests, hobbies, or causes. By preparing ahead of time, exhibiting flexibility, and being present, we may enjoy ourselves and our time with others.

Part III

The Variety of Connections

Chapter 11

Relationships differentiation in different environments and civilizations.

Cultural Variations in Relationships.

What are your thoughts on romantic, familial, and friend relationships? Have you ever considered how your cultural background has shaped the way you see these kinds of relationships? The truth is that cultural differences have a big influence on our relationships, as well as how we see and handle them.

Cultural Variations in the Significance of Relationships.

Although there are many factors that make us unique, cultural differences may have a significant effect on our social interactions. Relationship cultural variations distinguish us in our attitudes, beliefs, and values. They may influence a person's approach to relationships as well as how they manifest in cross-cultural interactions. Furthermore, our perception of what is normal or abnormal, good or wrong, might be influenced by cultural variances. These guidelines, which are also known as social standards, have a big influence on relationships.

Societal norms: appropriate conduct that complies with societal standards.

Every culture sets social standards or laws that all members of the community are required to abide by. While social norms in certain cultures tend to be more rigid and obvious, those in others could be more pliable and nuanced. Either way, our social connections are often affected by these cultural variations in social standards.

It is considered impolite to go to someone's house for supper and not finish everything on your plate in Layla's culture.

It's crucial to remember that relationships within cultures can vary based on culture. These subcultures might be associated with an area, religion, or economic standing.

Cultural Variations in the Psychology of Relationships

Individualist vs. collectivist cultures are a common lens through which psychologists analyze cultural variations in relationships.

Groups that put individual aims ahead of collective goals are said to be individualistic.

Groups that put collective objectives ahead of individual ones are said to be collectivist.

These two viewpoints significantly influence how cultural disparities in relationships are formed.

Cultural Differences' Effect on Relationships

Cultural variations may affect friendships and childrearing, among other social ties.

✦ Raising Children

When it comes to parenting children, cultural disparities in relationships may be particularly noticeable. Certain cultures mostly Western ones may place high importance on a child's independence and urge them to "be true to yourself" or "follow your heart."

On the other hand, other cultures emphasize obedience above all else.

Other cultures, like the Guise community in western Kenya, place greater emphasis on physical touch than on face-to-face communication in the parent-child bond. Others, like Senegal, forbid parents from conversing with young children. Conversely, Western societies may encourage constant conversation with children and fewer physical touch interactions, such as pushing a stroller. We cannot claim that one culture is superior to another despite these distinctions.

＋ Ties with friends

When it comes to friendships, cultural disparities in relationships become evident. Consider your perspective on friendships. Do you really believe that everyone on the planet shares your opinion of them? Or even think about your parents. Do they have any different perspectives on friendship than you do?

Though friendships take diverse forms and are seen differently in different cultures, they exist in all of them. For instance, Americans tend to have more friends with more disparities between them than those from other countries. Other cultures, such as Ghana, approach friendships with more caution (Adams & Plant, 2003). Certain cultures place a strong emphasis on the closeness and quality of their friendships.

How about friendships that conform to each other? Do some cultures have a higher risk of this than others?

Conformity is the act of altering one's thoughts and actions to meet the expectations of the group.

Yes, that is the response! Individualists are less likely to comply than persons from collectivist societies, according to research by Bond and Smith (1996). Do you have any theories as to why that may be?

+ Romantic Relationships

There might be significant cultural disparities in love relationships. Certain cultures could have very rigid and defined gender roles in romantic relationships.

Behaviors or characteristics that are socially expected of men or women are referred to as gender roles.

Furthermore, cultural perspectives on same-sex love partnerships might vary, and some may even have discriminatory legislation against LGBTQ+ people. Even the way that different cultures see interracial partnerships varies; some are more accepting than others. Cultural differences may provide particular difficulties for interracial couples as well as for their families, which can strain relationships.

Examples of Cultural Disparities in Relationships.

What are some concrete instances that you can think of when cultural differences affect your relationships? Do they stand out the most among friends, at school, or among strangers? Let's examine a few instances of how cultural differences might manifest in interpersonal interactions.

People are often more formal with strangers in non-American cultures than they are in North American societies.

Managing Relationship Cultural Differences.

It may be difficult to manage cultural differences in relationships in certain respects. Particularly in romantic relationships, this may be the case. How then do we handle these distinctions? It may ultimately boil down to how eager we are to work together. It does not always follow that you are right and they are incorrect just because your cultural values vary from someone else's. Every partner in a relationship has to be open to hearing the other person out. How can you make an effort to comprehend the perspective of the other person?

Open communication is another strategy we may use to address cultural differences in relationships. If no one discusses the topic in an open manner, how can we know there is a problem or difference of opinion? Open communication may aim to better comprehend one another's differences and create a common ground rather than necessarily changing the other person's opinion.

Chapter 12

Relationships evolution throughout the course of a person's life and developmental phases

Depending on our needs and talents in terms of the physical, cognitive, emotional, and social domains, relationships might alter as we mature. Relationships may alter in a number of ways as people age and go through developmental phases, including:

- Infancy: At this age, attachment and trust serve as the key pillars of partnerships. Because their caretakers offer them protection, comfort, and excitement, infants develop close relationships with them. Along with learning to express and understand emotions, infants also begin interacting with other people, such as siblings, relatives, or classmates.

- Childhood: Relationships at this age are mostly built on inquiry and education. Children want independence and autonomy from their caretakers as they grow in self-awareness and identity. Children who have similar interests, pastimes, and morals may also become buddies. Youngsters pick up social skills like cooperation, communication, and dispute resolution.

- Adolescence: Intimacy and identity are the primary building blocks of relationships throughout this time. Adolescents go through emotional, mental, and physical transitions as they try to define their own identities and place in the world. Teenagers may also develop romantic connections with other teenagers, who can provide them with support, tenderness, and love. Peer pressure, social comparison, and identity uncertainty are among the issues that adolescents face.

- Adulthood: Commitment and generativity serve as the primary foundations for partnerships at this period. Adults define their responsibilities in the home, workplace, and society while working for their objectives. In addition, adults have romantic connections with their spouses, who provide them stability, affection, and company. Transitions in life, including marriage, parenting, divorce, or retirement, can affect adults.

- Older adulthood: At this point, honesty and discernment are the primary building blocks of partnerships. As they age, people contemplate their past experiences and look for direction and significance in their lives. In addition, older persons continue to have interactions with their family and friends, who provide them emotional closeness, social support, and happy memories. Losses that older persons face include the passing of a loved one, deteriorating health, and social isolation.

Chapter 13

Relationships variation throughout categories and areas

"Relationship differentiation across types and domains" refers to the fact that relationships may take on different shapes and forms depending on the type of connection and the environment in which they are found. Relationships of all kinds, whether they be romantic, familial, friendship, or professional, have different goals, dynamics, and traits. A relationship's character and expectations are further influenced by the environment or domain in which it takes place, whether that setting is personal or professional. It basically refers to the many ways that relationships might change according to the kind of connection and the setting in which it occurs.

Consider how various sports relate to relationships:

Every sport has its own set of regulations, objectives, and methods of play.

Relationships are no different.

These are a few instances:

- Family relationships: Despite differences, you support and care for each other, much like a close-knit team.

Friendships: Sharing laughter and experiences with a friend while playing a game is a great way to spend time together.

- Romantic relationships: These are extraordinary partnerships in which you and a particular someone share profound emotions, aspirations, and ambitions.

- Work relationships: Similar to working with others in a project team, where you appreciate each other's abilities and work together to accomplish common objectives.

- Business relationships: Similar to negotiating a win-win scenario with a partner, when products or services are exchanged.

Key distinctions to keep in mind:

- Your objectives: Different relationship types have distinct objectives, such as love in romantic partnerships, success in professional connections, or financial gain in commercial relationships.

- Who's in charge: Power relationships may take many different forms, such as equal partners in a firm or parents mentoring children in a family.

How close you get: There are differences in the degree of intimacy; romantic and familial ties tend to be the most intimate, whilst professional interactions may be more formal.

- How you talk: Depending on the relationship, communication methods might vary, ranging from informal conversations with friends to formal emails with coworkers.

Relationship types and domains range greatly from one another because of the characteristics, setting, and intent behind each relationship. The following are some significant ways that connections vary across different kinds and domains:

1. The Relationship's Nature:

- Romantic Relationships:

- Marked by a romantic or sexual relationship and emotional closeness and affection.

Relationships with Family:

- Consists of biological or legal relatives, including parents, siblings, kids, and other family members.

- Friends:

- Built on a feeling of kinship, shared experiences, and common interests.

Relationships with Professions:

- Developed in a corporate or work environment, with an emphasis on reaching objectives.

2. Aims and Objectives:

- Love Partnerships:

- Mainly focused on friendship, emotional support, and creating a life together.

Relationships with Family:

- Frequently based on fostering, emotional support, and preserving family ties.

- Friends:

- Designed to foster friendship, common interests, and reciprocal personal development.

Relationships with Professions:

- Focused on teamwork, professional growth, and reaching shared objectives in the workplace.

3. Dedication and Anticipations:

- Love Partnerships:

- Frequently entail more emotional commitment and exclusivity demands.

Relationships with Family:

- Defined by expectations of assistance, family responsibilities, and a lifetime commitment.

- Friends:

- Involve different degrees of dedication according to the length and intensity of the friendship.

Relationships with Professions:

- Guided by the attainment of common goals, professional obligations, and competency standards.

4. Stability and Length:

- Love Partnerships:

- Can range greatly in length from casual dates to committed relationships.

Relationships with Family:

Although they are often seen of as lifetime relationships, stability may vary depending on personal circumstances.

- Friends:

- Vary from passing acquaintances to durable friendships that last a lifetime.

Relationships with Professions:

- May be short-term for particular projects or long-term for continuing professional cooperation.

5. Constitution and Willingness:

- Love Partnerships:

- Usually developed via mutual selection and attraction.

Relationships with Family:

Involuntary, often derived from birth or links to the law.

- Friends:

- On the basis of compatibility and same interests, voluntary contacts were made.

Relationships with Professions:

- Usually developed in a work environment, often based on duties and obligations of jobs.

6. Dynamis and Roles:

- Love Partnerships:

- Partners may adopt responsibilities-sharing positions like those of spouses or life partners.

Relationships with Family:

- Involves a variety of roles, each with unique dynamics, such as parents, siblings, and children.

- Friends:

- Roles are often more amorphous and determined by shared interests and unique personalities.

Relationships with Professions:

In a professional context, roles are determined by employment positions, responsibilities, and hierarchies.

7. Statement of Closeness:

- Love Partnerships:

- Require a great deal of closeness, both physically and emotionally.

Relationships with Family:

- Incorporate emotional connection and support; physical proximity may differ.

- Friends:

- Have less physical closeness overall, but may contain emotional intimacy as well.

Relationships with Professions:

- Consist primarily of a degree of professional intimacy, cooperation, and teamwork.

8. Delimitations:

- Love Partnerships:

- Emotional and personal space is often the focus of boundaries.

Relationships with Family:

- Boundaries may be complicated, including characteristics that are both family and personal.

- Friends:

- Boundaries are often flexible and predicated on mutual comprehension.

Relationships with Professions:

- Boundaries are usually established by duties and tasks in the workplace.

9. Results of Outside Factors:

- Love Partnerships:

- Social expectations, cultural standards, and legal concerns are examples of external variables.

Relationships with Family:

- Influenced by social standards, cultural expectations, and familial customs.

- Friends:

- Social networks, cultural influences, and personal situations are examples of external forces.

Relationships with Professions:

- Affected by the demands of society, industry norms, and workplace culture.

Knowing these distinctions helps you:

- Create stronger connections: You can make relationships more effective and meaningful by adjusting your behavior and expectations to fit each kind of relationship.

- Navigate various situations: Whether it's a family get-together, a business transaction, or a meeting at work, you'll know how to behave properly in various social contexts.

Chapter 14

How inclusion and diversity may improve relationships

The ideals of diversity and inclusion encourage tolerance and admiration for the many qualities and characteristics that make each person unique, including their gender, race, sexual orientation, ability, culture, and religion. Relationships may benefit from diversity and inclusion in a number of ways, including:

- Strengthening emotional intelligence and personal development: Being exposed to many cultures, viewpoints, and experiences may extend our views and increase our empathy. We may improve our interpersonal and communication abilities as well as learn more about ourselves and others. We may also confront our prejudices and preconceptions in order to broaden our horizons and increase our tolerance1.

- Creating an environment that is creative and innovative: People with diverse backgrounds and experiences may contribute a variety of perspectives, expertise, and abilities, which can lead to the development of fresh concepts and solutions. Diversity and inclusion may also create teamwork and synergy, as individuals can exploit their strengths and complement one another's weaknesses.

- Increasing satisfaction and performance: We may feel happier and more content when we are surrounded by people who appreciate, respect and support us. Diversity and inclusion can do this. Because there will be more possibilities and resources available to us to fulfill our dreams, diversity, and inclusion may also increase our motivation and productivity.

1. Wider Viewpoints:

- Diverse Backgrounds: Accepting diversity unites people with different opinions, life experiences, and cultural backgrounds.

- Enriched Conversations: Diverse perspectives provide for deeper conversations that deepen everyone's comprehension of a range of topics.

2. Enhanced Problem-Solving Skills:

- Diverse Skill Sets: Members of inclusive teams come from a variety of backgrounds and specializations.

- Collaborative issue solutions: Different viewpoints may result in more thorough approaches to issue solutions.

3. Enhanced Possibilities for Learning:

- Cultural Exchange: Diversity offers the chance to discover new customs, traditions, and civilizations.

- Skill Enhancement: People may learn from one another and acquire new skills when they are exposed to a variety of talents and skills.

4. Skill in Culture:

- Awareness Differences: By encouraging tolerance and awareness of differences, inclusive interactions enhance cultural competency.

- Decreased Stereotyping: Various viewpoints may dispel preconceptions and encourage more accurate views.

5. Enhanced Compassion:

- Shared Experiences: Being included promotes the sharing of individual narratives and life events.

- Building Empathy: Experiencing a variety of life situations increases empathy and a better understanding of the struggles and victories faced by others.

6. Fortifies Social ties:

- Common Values: Although diverse settings often emphasize common values like equality, opcnncss, and respect.

- Building Trust: People from diverse backgrounds might feel more at ease and connected in inclusive environments.

7. Self Development:

- Challenging Perspectives: Socializing with a variety of people dispels stereotypes and promotes personal development.

Adaptability: Being exposed to a variety of situations improves one's capacity for adjustment and for navigating various social and cultural environments.

8. Enhanced Performance and Productivity:

- Varied Skillsets: Diverse teams often provide a variety of complementary abilities.

Motivation: A more inclusive workplace may boost employees' drive and sense of fulfillment at work, which can enhance output.

9. International Viewpoint:

- International Collaboration: People may have global experiences and viewpoints in a variety of settings.

- International Networks: Global cooperation and commercial prospects may benefit from having access to a varied network.

10. Promotes Diversity Without Limitations:

- Emphasize Shared objectives: Inclusive partnerships often place a strong emphasis on shared values and objectives.

Reduced Bias: Making a concerted effort to promote inclusiveness lessens prejudices and fosters a more hospitable environment.

11. Building the Community:

- Community Engagement: Building a diverse and inclusive community is facilitated by connections.

Social Impact: Diverse people may work together to promote inclusiveness and constructive social change.

Chapter 15

Technology and Relationships.

Social media and technology have completely changed how we interact, connect, and sustain relationships.

Relationships may grow and develop in the following ways with the help of various digital platforms:

1. International Linkage:

- Cross-Cultural Connections: Through technology, people may communicate with others throughout the globe, promoting cross-cultural interactions.

- International Friendships: Social networking sites make it possible for friendships to grow across international borders.

2. Preserving Relationships Over Long Distances:

- Communication Tools: Social media, video calls, and instant messaging allow for real-time communication, which makes it simpler to maintain relationships with loved ones.

- Shared Experiences: People may feel more connected even when they are physically apart thanks to virtual platforms that facilitate sharing experiences.

3. Professional Networking Opportunities:

- Professional Networking: Websites such as LinkedIn provide chances to grow professional networks and build connections relevant to careers.

- Community Engagement: People may interact with like-minded persons and take part in a variety of online groups by using social media.

4. Establishing New Friendships:

- Social Media Platforms: People may strengthen and rekindle ties by connecting with old friends and acquaintances via websites like Facebook.

- Digital Memories: Posting pictures and recollections online fosters a sentimental connection with the past.

5. Updates in Real Time:

- Life Updates: People may keep updated on each other's lives by using social media platforms, which provide a constant flow of information about friends and relatives.

- Event Notifications: Thanks to technology, significant life events may be instantly announced, encouraging prompt and encouraging reactions.

6. Teamwork Projects:

- Virtual Collaboration: Whether for professional, leisure, or artistic purposes, technology facilitates teamwork on projects.

- Online Platforms: Programs like Google Drive or group editing software make it easier to collaborate and build connections.

7. Enhanced Interaction:

- Multimedia Communication: In addition to writing, people may communicate more deeply by exchanging images, videos, and voice messages.

- Immediate replies: Instant messaging promotes an immediate feeling of communication by enabling prompt replies.

8. Dating and Developing Relationships:

- Online Dating: Thanks to numerous platforms, technology makes the beginning phases of dating easier by enabling people to interact based on common interests.

- Virtual Dates: Online games and video chats provide substitutes for traditional dating and relationship development.

9. Friendly Communities:

- Online Support Groups: Thanks to technology, people with similar problems may interact and exchange experiences in encouraging groups.

- Mental Health Platforms: Online and app platforms provide areas for mental health resources and emotional support.

10. Learning and Development of Skills:

- Online Learning: Thanks to technology, people may take courses together to improve their skills and further their knowledge, resulting in shared learning opportunities.

- Virtual Workshops: Attending online workshops promotes a feeling of belonging and mutual development.

11. Coordination and Planning of Events:

- Invitations and organizing: Technology makes social ties stronger by streamlining the planning, sending out, and organizing of events.

- Virtual Events: Online get-togethers and events provide chances to socialize even in difficult or distant situations.

12. Communicative Inclusion:

Accessibility: Technology facilitates communication and encourages inclusion in relationships by making it easier for people with impairments to communicate.

- Translation Services: By using translation technologies, communication may be expanded across linguistic boundaries.

Conclusion

We have examined the impact of relationships on our happiness and well-being in this book, using data from science, anecdotes, and real-world guidance. We now know that relationships are essential to our physical, mental, and emotional well-being in addition to being a source of happiness and pleasure. Additionally, we now know that relationships are dynamic and ever-evolving and need ongoing care and attention. I hope that this book has improved both the quality and quantity of your social connections and has helped you see the worth and significance of your relationships. I hope that this book has inspired you to reach out to those who could benefit from your friendship or support and to widen your sphere of understanding and compassion. Partnerships are essential to people's pleasure and well-being they are not a luxury.

Regardless of age, gender, culture, or origin, I think everyone has a right to enjoy the advantages of fulfilling partnerships. Relationships are a talent and a decision that can be learned and practiced, not something that is determined by luck or destiny. Relationships are a mutually beneficial exchange of love and respect rather than a one-way path. Relationships are a reality that may result in happily ever after, not a fantasy.

Thank you for reading, kindly drop a review if you have enjoyed this book.

9 7 9 8 8 7 4 2 9 7 1 3 8